Hope Is Contagious

The Breast Cancer Treatment

Survival Handbook

Compiled by Margit Esser Porter

A FIRESIDE BOOK

Published by Simon & Schuster

F I R E S I D E
Rockefeller Center
1230 Avenue of the Americas, New York, NY 10020
Copyright © 1997 by Margit Esser Porter
All rights reserved, including the right of reproduction in whole
or in part in any form.

FIRESIDE and colophon are registered trademarks of Simon & Schuster Inc.

Designed by J Porter & Doreen Means

Manufactured in the United States of America
1 3 5 7 9 10 8 6 4 2
Library of Congress Cataloging-in-Publication Data
Porter, Margit Esser.
Hope is contagious: the breast cancer treatment survival handbook /
compiled by Margit Esser Porter.
p.   cm.
"A Fireside book."
1. Breast—Cancer—Patients—Quotations.
2. Breast—Cancer—Patients—Attitudes. 3. Questionnaires. I. Title.
RC280.B8P665 1997
362.1'9699449—dc21   97-23751
ISBN 0-684-84218-1   CIP

Dedication

THIS BOOK IS DEDICATED

to all the lupine ladies who sow the

seeds of wellness making the world a

more beautiful place, and to Aimee Hyatt,

for giving the seeds a place to grow.

Contents

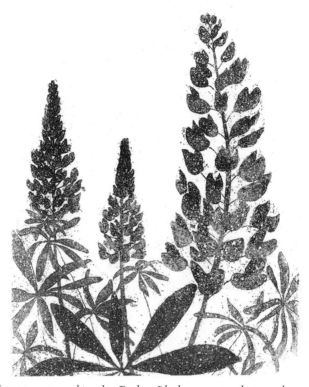

— LUPINES, *etching by Evelyn Rhodes, age 49, diagnosed 1990*

On May 18, 1980,

an earthquake triggered the eruption of Mount St. Helen's in Washington State. An area 24 miles square was destroyed, buried under 150 feet of ash, mud and rock. Scientists predicted the region would remain a dead zone for decades to come. Five years later a solitary lupine, blooming at the base of the mountain, proves them wrong. This is perhaps the most extraordinary of all earth's wonders: the ability to regenerate, to move on, to create anew.

— *LIFE* MAGAZINE, "EARTH'S WONDERS"

Hope Is
Contagious

Foreword

AT THE AGE OF 34, Margit Esser Porter learned that she had breast cancer. It is something she feared throughout her entire adult life, because her mother had discovered that she had breast cancer at the age of 35. Even the location of the tumor was the same —in the upper outer portion of her right breast. Margit went through every emotional response possible, even relief that what she feared had actually happened at last, and she had questions, millions of questions. She read everything available, rationalized, intellectualized, and suffered severe ups and downs. She vowed that she would not lose control of her mind or body. She also vowed that she would help other women through this incredibly difficult ordeal.

Margit fulfilled that vow by polling others who had experienced this life crisis, and compiling their responses, in their own words, in this book. These women reveal the things that they learned that would be of most help to others. Some insights are humorous and some are serious, but all are helpful.

What Margit has accomplished in *Hope Is Contagious* is a personal, informed, and compassionate book for women who have heard these words: "Your tumor is malignant." Using the experience and honesty of women who share a dreadful bond, the book responds to the questions and fears the diagnosis elicits: What will happen now? Will I be disfigured? Has my cancer spread? What kind of life lies ahead for me? What about my daughters? What changes must I make in my lifestyle?

No one can answer these questions better than the group of women Margit has polled. Here is a handbook that doesn't avoid hard truths, but that also is realistically hopeful and upbeat.

For the 185,000 women diagnosed with breast cancer annually in the United States, this handbook is just what the doctor ordered. I hope its readership will be wide, because the information in it is of inestimable value.

—NORMAN L. SADOWSKY, M.D.
Director of the Faulkner-Sagoff Breast Imaging and Diagnostic Centre

Introduction

"TAKE AN ACTIVE PARTICIPATION in your own survival." That's what my river guide advised as we put in the Colorado River of the Grand Canyon and prepared for the white water that lay ahead. He could never have known at the time that these would become words I lived by only four months later, after the diagnosis of my breast cancer and the class-10 rapids the treatment would bring.

One out of eight women gets breast cancer. That means that upon diagnosis, I instantly became a member of a group of women commonly regarded as a statistic, a number, an epidemic. I would bring to this group my own personal history, fears, feelings, and baggage, yet the treatment for this disease would basically be whatever protocol was statistically appropriate for the characteristics of my tumor. Everyone's cancer is unique. Everyone's situation is unique. I was, and still am, very much more than a number. I am an individual, a person, a woman.

This book is written by and for women who have had, and are going through, the treatment for breast cancer. It is to help you feel like something other than a number or a statistic. It is to help make your life simpler and more comfortable. The book is not written by M.D.s or Ph.D.s. The only authority we have to write this book is that we all have honorary degrees in tenacity and survival. The market is flooded with volumes about individual cases of breast cancer told in first-person dramatic narrative. I found these to be overwhelming. The last thing I wanted to do when I was diagnosed was read a dramatic account of some stranger's personal bout with near death. All I wanted was for someone to tell me how to get through it as quickly, simply, and comfortably as possible.

Hundreds of women have contributed suggestions that may help you through your treatment. This book is simply a survival reference handbook with some helpful ideas. It contains ideas your doctors may not tell you because they're too busy saving your life to be bothered with the "trauma" factor. I hope this helps you ride out the rapids and find your way back to happy trails.

In the back of the book you will find the questionnaire that was used to put together this book. Please help us keep updated by filling it out and sending it in after your treatment is completed. It is my goal to keep up the chain of women helping women.

Thanks and breast wishes!
MARGIT ESSER PORTER

Chapter One

Diagnosis

"Plan on a whopping phone bill. Don't
worry about paying it until later!"

— CHRISTY, *age 44, diagnosed 1995*

"There's something about breast cancer that makes it different from foot cancer or, for that matter, any other disease. It's about body image, it's about nurturing—it certainly is about femininity. It is loaded for women in ways that other health threats are not."

> — *Executive director of the National Alliance*
> *of Breast Cancer Organizations,*
> AMY S. LANGER, *age 42, diagnosed 1984*

"Although they don't have a cure yet, there are many new aggressive methods available. Go to a well-known hospital or clinic. Get two opinions. Then follow through with the program that was set up for you."

> — ALICE, *age 67, diagnosed 1980*

22

"Make sure that you're comfortable with your doctors. Once you are satisfied with your choice, don't let anyone undermine your confidence in the decisions that you make."

— CINDY, *age 42, diagnosed 1993*

"When I was diagnosed with breast cancer, I had these horrible anxiety attacks. I couldn't sleep and lost nine pounds in two weeks. I didn't want to take a prescription drug to relax, so I did some research and found a wonderful herb called valerian. Valerian drops in my water helped me get some sleep and some peace, without any side effects or loss of control."

— MARGIT, *age 35, diagnosed 1995*

"The best support I got was from a woman who had lived through both breast and ovarian cancer and was now 80 years old! My advice is to connect with women who have been there and are well now. Especially well in spirit!"

— PATRICIA, *age 53, diagnosed 1991*

"Instead of planning your death, plan your vacation. The pharmacy bills, hotel bills, phone bills, wigs, turbans, and prosthesis all add up. Charge it on one of those mileage-saving frequent-flier credit cards, and by the end of the arduous months of treatment there will be enough points for a free vacation! It's nice to have something to look forward to!"

— MARGIT, *age 35, diagnosed 1995*

"My husband had difficulty accepting my diagnosis. He went for counseling for the first time in his life, which ended up helping out both of us!"

— LINDY, *age 47, diagnosed 1984*

"Don't give up; inform yourself about the disease and be honest about it to others."

— RUTH, *age 74, diagnosed 1984*

"I had always thought that a diagnosis of breast cancer meant having to lose a breast. I was so relieved to find out that these days in many cases you can keep your breast and not have to trade it in for your life."

— SARAH, *age 29, diagnosed 1994*

"I believe that there are at least as many 'so-so' doctors out there as there are really good ones—find the one that works for and with you!"

— LINDY, *age 47, diagnosed 1984*

"I got support from my faith in God."

— EMMA, *age 67, diagnosed 1995*

"I learned a key survival skill from my golden retriever when he developed cataracts in both of his eyes. Cataracts, unlike cancer, are not life threatening, but they can affect one's quality of life. My dog still plays like a puppy because he has learned to see with his nose."

— MARGIT, *age 35, diagnosed 1995*

"Get support from family and friends, but research the disease as much as you possibly can."

— JOANNE, *age 50, diagnosed 1990*

"I got support from three close friends who maintained constant contact with me. All three had breast cancer."

— LOIS, *age 50, diagnosed 1994*

"If you work, keep working. If you have a social life, keep socializing. Don't let the cancer downgrade your life. Rather, force it into a role of enhancing your life. "

— BETTE, *age 45, diagnosed 1985 & 1995*

"Don't let today's trial bog you down. Think of it as a long process where you win at the end."

— EVELYN, *age 49, diagnosed 1990*

"My cancer was very early stage in situ. Most people would say that with such a diagnosis a mastectomy is ridiculous and totally unnecessary, but it's what I chose. It's my body, my life, and I'm the one living with the decision. I'm glad I did it and have no regrets."

— ANNETTE, *age 74, diagnosed 1988*

"My husband helped me by embarking on a major research mission."

— SHARON, *age 32, diagnosed 1996*

"I told people myself about my diagnosis because I found it helpful for people to hear the truth from me rather than gossip and speculation."

— CINDY, *age 42, diagnosed 1993*

"I knew I had to live for my husband and kids. No matter what lay ahead, I had to go through it so I could be around for them!"

— SUSAN, *age 38, diagnosed 1991*

"Go and get a flu shot if you get diagnosed in the fall. Treatment in the winter is hard enough without catching the flu!"

— BONITA, *age 39, diagnosed 1994*

"Shortly after my diagnosis, I saw an ad for The Susan G. Komen Breast Cancer Foundation's Race for the Cure. I called the foundation (see Resources, page 145) and got the date of a race scheduled in my area, to take place after the expected completion date of my treatment. Some friends thought I was setting myself up for disappointment. Others knew I was setting a goal for myself. I ran that race! My oncologist ran it with me and waited for me at the finish line with a smile and a sweaty hug!"

— MARGIT, *age 35, diagnosed 1995*

"I told everyone in my personal life, but not in my professional life."

— SANDY, *age 47, diagnosed 1995*

"If I stop and think about the future I get really frightened. Almost paralyzed. When this happens I force myself to go do something fun. I always do something that I never would have done before my diagnosis of breast cancer."

— JOAN, *age 30, diagnosed 1994*

"I lost my job because they said I no longer fit into their long-term goals. My new job is a much better one that I love."

— CONNIE, *age 41, diagnosed 1985, 1994, & 1996*

"Listen to music. Watch birds."

— GAIL, *age 49, diagnosed 1994*

"When I was diagnosed with breast cancer the first thing I did was go to talk with someone who put my head in the right place spiritually. With my head in the right place I knew I could take on anything!"

— ALICE, *age 42, diagnosed 1994*

"I had a really close friend who allowed me to call whenever I had one of my anxiety attacks. She talked me through them at all hours of the night."

— AMY, *age 40, diagnosed 1995*

"I got lots of cards and letters from the school where I work, which was wonderful support."

— GAIL, *age 49, diagnosed 1994*

"From the first day of diagnosis I had to learn to live with fear and the ambiguity of this disease. The not knowing has been harder than any of the treatments. I finally found a place for the constant uncertainty of breast cancer. I take chances I never took before. I live life one day at a time and savor every moment."

— ELIZABETH, *age 35, diagnosed 1995*

"I live alone and had a mastectomy and reconstruction with no support other than from my doctors. I managed to handle it myself. It's been ten years since my diagnosis of breast cancer."

— MARJORIE, *age 76, diagnosed 1986*

"My husband was endlessly loving, supportive, and helpful from the moment I was diagnosed right through treatment. He helped me laugh and fight and I couldn't have done it without him."

— JANET, *age 56, diagnosed 1993*

"My husband was too scared to support me, but my children were grown and I was happy about that."

— MARY, *age 70, diagnosed 1975*

"Get a 'big sister' who has been in your shoes and can talk you through treatment. Make sure she's close to you in age."

— BEVERLY, *age 53, diagnosed 1993*

"The doctors had a conference about my tumor, which was the size of a walnut and close to the chest wall. They told me I had one year to live. That was twenty-six years ago!"

— MARTHA, *age 74, diagnosed 1970*

"I was diagnosed the day before my wedding. My husband was, and still is, very supportive."

— JANE, *age 26, diagnosed 1994*

"I had a boyfriend who was not at all supportive. We broke up. I lost my breast, but I chose to give up my boyfriend."

— JULIE, *age 50, diagnosed 1985*

"I went to the library and read everything I could find about breast cancer."

— PATRICIA, *age 52, diagnosed 1985*

"There is loads of support out there for the taking. Look for and find it."

— HOLLY, *age 57, diagnosed 1983*

"Nobody but us really knows what it's like."

— *Television producer, journalist, author,*
LINDA ELLERBEE, *age 52, diagnosed 1992*

"Cry when you need to."

— ANNE, *age 57, diagnosed 1996*

"Not all cancers are the same. Each person's treatment may differ because of the type of disease. Talk, talk, talk."

— GAIL, *age 41, diagnosed 1994*

"It's a great time to encourage other women to get a mammogram."

— BETSY, *age 51, diagnosed 1995*

"I believe in eating a well-balanced diet with small helpings of a great variety of foods, watching one's weight, and sensible exercise. Enjoy yourself in this life!"

— *Author, teacher,*
JULIA CHILD, *age 85, diagnosed 1952*

"I never missed a day of work and found that it's what kept me going and where I got the most support."

— ALISON, *age 44, diagnosed 1994*

"My mother was a great source of support for me. She had breast cancer also."

— PAULA, *age 34, diagnosed 1995*

"Ask every question that comes into your mind and don't be shy about it. Doctors charge a great deal, so don't let them make you feel you're wasting their time with stupid questions. The unasked question is the only stupid one."

— BEVERLY, *age 32, diagnosed 1995*

"Be sure to bring a list of questions to the doctor's office. That way when you're nervous you won't forget them all. Also it's a good idea to bring someone with you to help interpret the answers and to write them down."

— MARIA, *age 47, diagnosed 1990*

"We live in an age when cancer no longer has to mean a death sentence."

— EDYTHE, *age 86, diagnosed 1996*

"What you do initially for treatment impacts your options down the road. Most women aren't told that."

— VIRGINIA, *age 45, diagnosed 1989 & 1991*

"I remember clearly the first time I laughed after the traumatic news of my diagnosis. It was when my friend Marilyn frantically called trying to help by telling me where I could get a ton of information about breast cancer. She told me about the National Cancer Institute's help line. I've always been a terrible speller so she clearly spelled it out for me. 1-800-4-C-A-N-C-E-R. The irony of this made me giggle uncontrollably."

— MARGIT, *age 35, diagnosed 1995*

"I took time off from work so I could pamper myself and deal with my diagnosis. I loved doing it but was sorry it took cancer for me to do this."

— SUE, *age 35, diagnosed 1994*

"Cancer survivorship is a topic of interest to almost everyone. We read that one in eight women will develop breast cancer—one in three will develop cancer in some form. No family is without its experience with this terrifying disease. My personal experience and observations are like those of others. When we are dealing with things as basic as life and death, there is a universality to the experience. We are all in this together. We need each other, and we need as much help as we can get to face and deal with cancer when it affects us or someone close to us."

— *United States Supreme Court Justice,*
SANDRA DAY O'CONNOR, *age 67, diagnosed 1988*

"Don't make decisions too quickly. If possible get more than one opinion."

— MARSHA, *age 55, diagnosed 1995*

"I was diagnosed with stage three B inflammatory breast cancer with ten positive nodes. I had a bone marrow transplant and the works, but got through it with the support of my friends, family, partner, and church."

— JUANITA, *age 29, diagnosed 1994*

"I did not associate with anyone who spoke negatively."

— LORRAINE, *age 56, diagnosed 1993*

"One of the things we did right away when I was diagnosed was to recognize the possible role chemicals (hormones in meats, pesticides and fungicides in produce, as well as additives and preservatives in most foods) may have played in the genetic changes that had to have taken place in my body for cancer to have grown. As a result, primarily for the sake of our daughters, we began an involved process of changing to an entirely natural organic diet from a typical American diet. Our home is now 95 percent organic, but we are flexible when eating out or at others' homes. At the time we made the change, it gave me an important sense of control over a world gone crazy for me, and hopefully will have a biological benefit for both of our girls."

— CINDY, *age 42, diagnosed 1993*

"My husband stayed beside me, holding my hand throughout every examination and visit. He was not willing to wait in the reception room. He always stated when asked that he needed to be a second pair of ears for his wife. He was right. When we would discuss the visits and what had been said, I invariably had heard only the negative side of each opinion. He remembered and reminded me of the positives."

— BARBARA, *age 73, diagnosed 1988*

"Don't read the statistics and put yourself in them. You are an individual with your own set of circumstances. Use the statistics as a guide, not a road map for your situation."

— CINDY, *age 40, diagnosed 1994*

"Once you get the diagnosis of breast cancer, don't be surprised if all your friends feel the need to give you their advice. They usually just want to help in some way, but because of the misconceptions surrounding the disease you may hear things that are overwhelming. I remember when a guy told me that I should be grateful because breast cancer was the best kind of cancer for a woman to get. I should have replied that prostate cancer was the best kind for a woman to get, but I was too blown away to respond."

— MARGIT, *age 35, diagnosed 1995*

"Let people do things for you. Friends and family usually want to help, so let them."

— PATRICIA, *age 37, diagnosed 1996*

"I did jigsaw puzzles. Each piece you put in is like rebuilding your life."

— AMY, *age 44, diagnosed 1995*

"If you don't already have one, get an answering machine. Your private life is about to become everyone's reason to reach out and touch you."

— EMILY, *age 54, diagnosed 1996*

"Be not afraid. Many women are living proof of survival with joy and many years ahead. Keep positive thoughts; look ahead eagerly and with hope!"

— ANNA, *age 74, diagnosed 1988*

"Hang on tight. It's a roller coaster for a while, but it does get better."

— EMILY, *age 47, diagnosed 1994*

"Read *Dr. Susan Love's Breast Book.*"

— BONNIE, *age 49, diagnosed 1992*

"If I had a choice, I would choose not to have breast cancer. But no one gave me that option, so I make use of this disease. I use it as a platform to mobilize all women and men to raise their voice to eradicate breast cancer. Join us!"

— *President of the National Breast Cancer Coalition,*
FRANCES M. VISCO, *age 49, diagnosed 1987*

Chapter Two

Surgery

"Wear comfy clothes to the hospital."

—CAROL, *age 61, diagnosed 1988*

"I have always been a needle phobic. Knowing that I had invasive cancer and was going to be treated with chemotherapy, I found it helpful that my doctor informed me about the option of having a venous access device implanted at the same time as my breast surgery. Kind of like one-stop shopping!"

— MARGIT, *age 35, diagnosed 1995*

"Up to the point of surgery, I had followed a regular exercise program based on swimming. After surgery and during chemo, I was unable to muster any extra energy for workouts. Yoga was the saving factor."

— EVELYN, *age 49, diagnosed 1990*

"I teach tennis for a living, and am able to keep doing so and play competitive tennis."

— SUE, *age 56, diagnosed 1988*

"The narcotics from surgery made me get nasty hemorrhoids. This caused big problems for me when I went through chemotherapy. My advice is to take a stool softener before and after surgery."

— ANN, *age 35, diagnosed 1995*

"The hospital gave me a little pillow to use under my arm where I had the mastectomy and removal of lymph nodes. It helped make me more comfortable."

— RUTH, *age 74, diagnosed 1984*

"I requested that my surgeries be first thing in the morning. That way, by the time I truly woke up, it would just be the time that I would normally start my day. For me this meant I wouldn't be sick from starvation and lack of thirst on top of the anesthesia."

— ALICE, *age 38, diagnosed 1996*

"Wear socks. It gets cold in the operating room."

— JOANNE, *age 33, diagnosed 1996*

"Buy a Bucky pillow to support your arm after surgery. They're wonderful!" (See Resources, page 145.)

— MARGIT, *age 35, diagnosed 1995*

"I requested that my surgery be early in the week. I didn't want to wait all weekend for the pathology report."

— ANN, *age 35, diagnosed 1995*

"Get good strong drugs. Now is no time to be brave!"
— HEATHER, *age 46, diagnosed 1994*

"Wear a soft cotton button-down shirt to the hospital. It's hard to lift your arm over your head immediately after the axillary dissection. I even slept in my husband's oxford button-down shirts!"

— EDITH, *age 39, diagnosed 1996*

"The weird thing about surgery is that after it's over, the hard part begins. With other illnesses, surgery is the entire treatment."

— ELLEN, *age 38, diagnosed 1995*

"After surgery, treat yourself to your favorite dessert."

— LISA, *age 30, diagnosed 1993 & 1996*

"If you have a lumpectomy you get to go home the same day. This is both a blessing and a curse. In the hospital they have visiting hours. Make sure you have someone around at home to keep away unwanted visitors."

— ROSE, *age 48, diagnosed 1994*

"Have your doctor whisper the words *clean margins* in your ear while you're under anesthesia. Can't hurt. Might help!"

— MARGIT, *age 35, diagnosed 1995*

"You can't eat or drink before surgery, but you can brush you teeth if you don't swallow any water. It's these little things that make you feel human."

— ALICE, *age 40, diagnosed 1996*

"When I had my lumpectomy, the surgery was about seventy minutes but the recovery room time was nearly two and a half hours!"

— LISA, *age 34, diagnosed 1995*

"The drains they put in hurt more than the mastectomy."

— BEVERLY, *age 47, diagnosed 1996*

"If you don't want a student to put in your intravenous line, make sure you speak up. As a cancer patient, you'll be getting enough needles. Let the students practice on the elective surgery cases; like those in for liposuction!"

— WENDY, *age 47, diagnosed 1996*

"My boyfriend came with me to all of my surgeries."

— LESLIE, *age 26, diagnosed 1995*

"If a test is missing or late, follow up. It may be lost. Don't assume it's just late."

— JANET, *age 56, diagnosed 1993*

"Your surgeon is only the first in your team of doctors helping you on the road to recovery. If it's at all possible, try to have all your doctors in the same hospital. That way, hopefully, they'll confer with each other and work as a team when treating you."

— JANE, *age 56, diagnosed 1992*

"My mastectomy surgery took nearly nine hours because I had reconstruction at the same time."

— ELLEN, *age 40, diagnosed 1993*

"When I went in for my first surgery I was scared to death. I was convinced that they'd put me to sleep and I'd never wake up again. (I must have seen the movie *Coma* one too many times.) By the time my third surgery came along, I was pretty relaxed and knew all the orderlies by name. I actually was excited about seeing my favorite recovery room nurse, M.J."

— MARGIT, *age 35, diagnosed 1995*

"Vacuum under the bed before you go to the hospital. Change the sheets too. There's nothing like coming home to a clean bed."

— CINDY, *age 42, diagnosed 1993*

"I had to give up swimming, tennis, and golf for a while, but I was able to walk every day."

— ELIZABETH, *age 35, diagnosed 1995*

"I still think it's a medicine tried and true, especially after surgery: chicken soup!"

— LOIS, *age 54, diagnosed 1995*

"I loved the fact that even though my doctor insisted I load up on protein before and after surgery, she never frowned upon my vegetarian diet. She just said that I should eat more protein, be it beans or tofu, sprouts or carrot juice; just as long as I ate protein. Lots of it!"

— MARGIT, *age 35, diagnosed 1995*

"My favorite food after surgery was warm oatmeal."

— ALICE, *age 44, diagnosed 1996*

"I used to get really sick from anesthesia, but these days they have great antiemetics. Gone are my days of waking up with a sore throat from the breathing tube, or an upset stomach from the drugs!"

— MARY, *age 42, diagnosed 1995*

"Don't take off or change your bandages when you're tired. If possible, have a friend or someone you're close with help you."

— EMILY, *age 46, diagnosed 1993*

"If you ever had a past reaction to anesthesia (good or bad), be sure to get hold of the records and show them to your anesthesiologist. That way, he or she can try to adjust the medication for your next surgery. It might prevent another bad experience or serve to duplicate a good one."

— LOIS, *age 54, diagnosed 1995*

"I kept finding heart monitoring tabs on my body for days after the surgery. They left sticky sore spots when I pulled them off. Have someone give you the once-over when you leave the hospital and get rid of the silly things!"

— SHARON, *age 32, diagnosed 1996*

"Right up to the point of going under from anesthesia, I listened, via headphones, to a relaxation tape that I brought with me to pre-op."

— SHARON, *age 32, diagnosed 1996*

"Go out to dinner and treat yourself to your favorite fattening food the night before surgery. You'll lose every pound the next day, so you may as well party till midnight."

— LISA, *age 34, diagnosed 1995*

"I wrote a list of healing statements for the anesthesiologist to read to me during surgery."

— SHARON, *age 32, diagnosed 1996*

"There's a drug they give you so that you won't remember anything from the moment they give it to you until when you wake up. I'm not kidding; it's amazing stuff. I'm told that I had entire conversations with nurses I swear I've never met!"

— MARY, *age 42, diagnosed 1995*

"If you've already had an axillary node dissection and you're back getting more surgery, don't let them take your blood pressure from the arm that's missing the lymph nodes. You could end up with lymphedema."

— JOAN, *age 30, diagnosed 1994*

"I prepared lots of food that I could freeze ahead of time so that when I got home from the hospital all I had to do for meals was heat and eat."

— DEBORAH, *age 42, diagnosed 1996*

"Some advice I encountered was to buy an electric shaver for my underarms so that I wouldn't nick the numb area after the axillary node dissection. I think this advice was given by someone who didn't think that a woman could be careful enough not to cut herself. I wasted money on an electric shaver that I never use. I use disposable razors and I never cut myself!"

— EVELYN, *age 49, diagnosed 1990*

"The effects of anesthesia last for weeks after surgery. Don't be upset if your energy level is a bit off for a while."

— LOIS, *age 54, diagnosed 1995*

"Friends from work made complete meals for me and my family and delivered them fresh each day for a week after I got home from the hospital. We never ate the same thing twice. It was a huge help for which I was truly grateful."

— ALISON, *age 44, diagnosed 1994*

"I started practicing meditation."

— LOIS, *age 50, diagnosed 1994*

"As soon as you are able, after surgery, start moving your arm around so you don't get a frozen shoulder."

— LISA, *age 34, diagnosed 1995*

"In the nine years since my initial diagnosis, I've had two recurrences, each time requiring surgery. After the last recurrence I joined a support group and have found it extremely helpful."

— KANA, *age 56, diagnosed 1987*

"Don't drink any green tea for a week before surgery. It's a natural blood thinner."

— JOAN, *age 30, diagnosed 1994*

"I think that the hardest part of my surgery was waiting for the pathology report to come back."

— DEBORAH, *age 42, diagnosed 1996*

"After my surgery, I got a visit in the hospital from a member of the Reach to Recovery program (see Resources, page 145). She was very supportive."

— SUE, *age 56, diagnosed 1988*

"Surgery doesn't always come first in the line of treatment. Sometimes it comes last. Maybe that's because, as the saying goes, they save the best for last."

— BEVERLY, *age 32, diagnosed 1995*

"For me activism was not a conscious decision. It just happened. I wrote my first article when I was in the hospital recovering from surgery. I had to keep telling nurses, aides, and doctors not to touch my compromised arm. It was then that I decided hospitals needed to identify this arm with a pink wrist band. Spread the word so that we can make this a national mandate! A pink band is a simple, effective tool that can help alert people to the risks regarding lymphedema!"

> — *Postal worker who spearheaded the campaign for*
> *the first Breast Cancer Awareness postage stamp,*
> DIANE SACKETT NANNERY, *age 44, diagnosed 1993*

"Make sure a nurse shows you what exercises you can and should do to help the side where you have your surgery."

— LILLIAN, *age 81, diagnosed 1996*

"After my breast surgery people kept asking me if it was my right breast that had the cancer or my left. Do you suppose if it had been a brain tumor they would have asked right lobe or left?"

— MARGIT, *age 35, diagnosed 1995*

Chapter Three

Chemotherapy

"I did my makeup each morning,
no matter how awful I felt, and it
helped me feel more normal."

— CINDY, *age 42, diagnosed 1993*

"It sucks in a major league way, but there are good antiemetics out there (like Zofran). You can do it, but expect good weeks, when you're strong, and bad weeks, when you'll need to baby yourself."

— CHRISTY, *age 44, diagnosed 1995*

"Just before starting my treatment with the drug Adriamycin, I did two things to my hair; first I had it cut off one inch from my head so I'd have an idea of what it might look like when it would start to grow back, and then I shaved it right down to the scalp. This gave me a sense of control, and instantly removed one of the side effects."

— MARGIT, *age 35, diagnosed 1995*

"When I started chemo I also started regular acupuncture sessions, meditation, and weekly massage treatments. I read many books, took walks on a regular basis, long warm baths, and accepted the support of coworkers and friends."

— LOIS, *age 50, diagnosed 1994*

"After each round of chemo I did not feel well for about three days. In that time I indulged myself and rested. Milk shakes soothed and comforted me."

— ANN, *age 68, diagnosed 1972 & 1991*

"I made a collage out of my hair."

— SHARON, *age 32, diagnosed 1996*

"I ate macaroni and cheese, applesauce, saltines, and yogurt."

— PATRICIA, *age 53, diagnosed 1988*

"The emotional roller coaster the drugs caused made me a bit 'crazy.' Some days I would be nearly euphoric, only to be met with brutal depression the next day. I kept a journal, and related the drugs I had taken and how I felt. This helped me to judge how my next treatment cycle might go and better plan when might or might not be a good day to see friends, etc. My dog became my shadow. She could read my emotional temperature and always seemed to know what to do."

— LINDY, *age 47, diagnosed 1984*

❧

"When my blood counts were low, I kept surgical masks by the front door for visitors. That way I didn't have to be isolated like a prisoner in my own home."

— SHARON, *age 32, diagnosed 1996*

"Mouth sores made eating difficult, so I drank a lot of protein drinks to keep my strength up."

— SYLVIA, *age 46, diagnosed 1997*

"I couldn't drink enough liquids, so I made frozen pops out of organic fruit juices and sucked on them to keep the fluids up."

— SHARON, *age 32, diagnosed 1996*

"I ate Black Mission figs to counteract constipation from the Zofran."

— SHARON, *age 32, diagnosed 1996*

"Make sure you find out everything you can about the long-term side effects of the chemotherapy that you sign up for. Particularly the damage to your immune system and bone marrow."

— LYNN, *age 35, diagnosed 1995*

"I nibbled on crackers all the time to keep the nausea at bay."

— JANET, *age 56, diagnosed 1993*

❧

"I have a hickman. I call it Mr. Hickman. It's the best thing ever. No more needles!"

— LISA, *age 30, diagnosed 1993 & 1996*

"My straight, fine hair grew back thick and wavy after I finished chemo. It was a great positive side effect. I tell people that I went to the hair club for women, and I refer to it as my $10,000 perm!"

— MARGIT, *age 35, diagnosed 1995*

"Don't let yourself get dehydrated while you're on chemo. Drink, drink, drink!"

— ELAINE, *age 53, diagnosed 1985*

❧

"I maintained my health club membership, even though I was too tired to use it."

— NICANDRA, *age 38, diagnosed 1994*

"I was on CMF. It made everything taste metallic, so I ate with plastic utensils."

— ELLA, *age 45, diagnosed 1995*

"There's a lot of information about chemotherapy and the various protocols on the Internet. My husband was very helpful because he accessed information for me via the Net."

— BETSY, *age 51, diagnosed 1995*

❧

"Wear bright colors. Stay away from grays, greens, and yellows."

— PATRICIA, *age 37, diagnosed 1996*

"I had a venous access device and found it very helpful! Unfortunately it had to be taken out because I developed a line infection."

— LYNN, *age 35, diagnosed 1995*

"I took a year off from teaching. Originally I planned to return in April at the end of chemo, but I was too exhausted to do it."

— RAYA, *age 60, diagnosed 1990*

"Get your teeth cleaned before you start chemo."

— HILLARY, *age 31, diagnosed 1994*

"I was given a lot of flowers and I enjoyed spending time arranging them. In the spring I worked in the garden."

— RAYA, *age 60, diagnosed 1990*

"The smell of any flower or perfume made me sick. The slightest sound, even the dripping of a faucet, made my head pound. The faintest glimmer of light made me wince and my sense of taste was totally altered. Thankfully, when chemo ended, that all went away."

— DIANE, *age 40, diagnosed 1995*

"Get a really good skin moisturizer and use it often."

— EMILY, *age 38, diagnosed 1996*

"Don't be afraid to cancel plans. There are good days and bad days, so don't force yourself to do something just because you said you would."

— SALLY, *age 60, diagnosed 1994*

"Chemo made everything taste salty to me."

— RITA, *age 42, diagnosed 1996*

"I got dressed every day even if I wasn't going to leave the house."

— RAYA, *age 60, diagnosed 1990*

"The only water I could drink that didn't taste metallic to me was bottled water. I also started craving poultry, which was really weird because I'm a vegetarian."

— SUSANNA, *age 35, diagnosed 1994*

"Spend time with your pet."

— LISA, *age 30, diagnosed 1993 & 1996*

"My eyes drove me nuts! They were dry and red all the time, which made me look like I had been crying. I found a wonderful over-the-counter eye moisturizer that didn't contain any preservatives called Thera Tears, which my eyes drank all day long."

— SUSAN, *age 53, diagnosed 1996*

"I had three children in their twenties when I went through chemo. I was very open with them about it and tried to answer all of their questions."

— BETSY, *age 51, diagnosed 1995*

"I wanted to maintain some sense of normalcy in the house for my two daughters. I didn't want their world to fall apart because of what I was going through. One thing that I made an effort to do was make certain that our family sat down together every night for dinner and I did my best to keep a normal routine around the house."

— CINDY, *age 42, diagnosed 1993*

"I gained a lot of weight and found that water reten-
tion was the problem."

— CHRISTINE, *age 58, diagnosed 1990*

"I hated losing my lashes and eyebrows. It was worse
than losing the hair on my head! "

— BECKY, *age 50, diagnosed 1996*

"My insurance was Blue Cross Blue Shield of New
Hampshire Managed Care. For two days each month after
my treatments, I was so sick that my husband was
afraid to go to work and leave me alone. At first he
took time off from work, and we also relied on friends.
I called B.C.B.S. of N.H., and asked if for two days each

month, they could provide in-home nursing. Even
though this was not covered in our policy, they not
only provided us with nursing care, but also assigned
a nutritionist to my case to make certain that I was
getting the proper food while undergoing treatment. The
insurance company and I agreed that it was to everyone's
benefit to keep me at home and out of the hospital,
where the bills would have been far more expensive than
a few days of in-home nursing care. Don't be afraid to
ask for help even if it's not in your policy."

— MARGIT, *age 35, diagnosed 1995*

"I drank ginger tea to settle my stomach."

— NANCY, *age 43, diagnosed 1993*

"Try to remember that there are other things going on in your life. Don't just focus on the moment."

— ROSE, *age 46, diagnosed 1988*

"Going back into chemotherapy after you've had a break from it for a while requires some heavy mind/ body discipline. I saw a specialist in this field so she could help me go back to the hospital. Her main advice was to change the way I had chemo adminis- tered. Have it in a different room. Bring some orange oil to the hospital so the smell of the place was differ- ent. She even suggested that I wear different clothing to my treatments and ask for a different nurse to administer the drugs."

— SHARON, *age 32, diagnosed 1996*

"Everyone fears the chemo bald look. First off, not all chemo drugs make you lose all of your hair. Second of all, if you do lose it, there are some advantages like the low maintenance, the coolness in summer, and seeing your gorgeous face and shape of your head without the distraction of hair. Last of all, know this ... *It does grow back!*"

— EMILY, *age 42, diagnosed 1996*

"The effects of the drugs were definitely cumulative. Each time I went in for a treatment it took me a bit longer to rebound."

— JACQUELINE, *age 46, diagnosed 1996*

"While on chemo, I ice-skated every Saturday for three hours."

— BARBARA, *age 52, diagnosed 1992*

"I view chemotherapy as just one of my aids to help me meet the challenge of breast cancer. Believing in the treatment makes it easier to get through."

— LAURA, *age 60, diagnosed 1997*

"While I was undergoing chemotherapy, my husband joined a support group for spouses. Because he found a way to deal with his feelings, he was better able to help me."

— DENISE, *age 58, diagnosed 1997*

"I was not one to wear much makeup before I had chemo, so I didn't wear much while in treatment. The void where I had once had bushy eyebrows was too obvious to let go unpainted, so I did put on eyebrow powder each day. I found powder was much more natural looking than pencil."

— MARIANNE, *age 36, diagnosed 1996*

"Try to find the positive in each step of your treatment. You've joined (though unwillingly) a group of very courageous, remarkable women. Learn from them. Let them help you get through this difficult time and then you can help others get through it."

— SUSAN, *age 53, diagnosed 1996*

"By the first round of chemo, even my dogs knew I had cancer."

— MARGIT, *age 35, diagnosed 1995*

"It's hard to sleep when you're nauseated, and I hated not sleeping. I consulted with a naturopath who tried to help me unoverwhelm my liver with herbal concoctions and hot compresses on the liver at bedtime. It seemed to help a little."

— CINDY, *age 42, diagnosed 1993*

"I had CMF and it didn't stop me from walking two miles a day, five days a week."

— JANE, *age 51, diagnosed 1995*

"I liked to suck on ice cubes while the chemo drugs were being administered into my intravenous line."

— MAUREEN, *age 44, diagnosed 1993*

"Think of chemo as an anatomy lesson. You're about to discover all of the places mucous membranes live in your body, because when they vacate, you'll know it! This is my chemo shopping list to help with the side effects of missing mucous membranes: baking soda (to gargle with and keep mouth sores at bay), hemorrhoidal ointment, comfrey salve, vaginal lubricating cream, anti-fungal cream, a laxative, and a good unscented moisturizing cream for every part of your body."

— JULIA, *age 33, diagnosed 1996*

"Everyone tells me to try to keep a positive attitude. Is that supposed to help me or them? I'm taking poison! Let's reality test, please!"

— JULIA, *age 33, diagnosed 1996*

"To combat the nausea, I ate little bits of food all day long instead of three meals a day."

— TRUDI, *age 38, diagnosed 1996*

"About halfway through my treatment I became very depressed and had to go on antidepressants so that I could complete my chemo. I also started power walking. Both things helped a great deal."

— SANDY, *age 47, diagnosed 1995*

"When people ask me why I'm not trying alternative treatments I tell them the following: When I was diagnosed at the age of 34 with a highly prolific, infiltrating, poorly differentiated breast tumor, I had been what my cousin the doctor had jokingly referred to as a skinny, nondrinking, nonsmoking, homeopathic, vegetarian jock. None of those titles kept me from getting breast cancer. For me, Western medicine, especially chemotherapy, is alternative treatment."

— MARGIT, *age 35, diagnosed 1995*

"Wear big earrings and enjoy the shape of your raw head!"

— SHARON, *age 32, diagnosed 1996*

"I kept hearing from women about how much weight
I'd gain on chemo. I lost weight and it wasn't for lack
of eating."

— ALICE, *age 34, diagnosed 1996*

"Before you get fed up with inexperienced nurses trying to draw your blood from veins that have long given
up, protect yourself! Request to have your blood
drawn by a phlebotomist. That's all they do, and they
usually do it much better than even the most experienced nurse!"

— EMILY, *age 42, diagnosed 1996*

"I did well because my doctors and the hospital staff believed in me and in the stem cell program. I will always be grateful for what they did. My life will never be the same, but after 18 months of fighting for life, I am still alive, and I can finally see the end of treatment!"

— MARJORIE, *age 42, diagnosed 1995*

"The hardest part of chemo for me was having to take the chemo drugs by pill each day. I would have preferred a protocol where a nurse gave me all the drugs by intravenous all at once. At least then I wouldn't have had to feel like I was poisoning myself."

— LOUISA, *age 48, diagnosed 1996*

"I was close to natural menopause, so I wasn't surprised when chemotherapy induced it for me. Other women told me that eating soy products might help with hot flashes, so I ate my morning cereal with soy milk. It seemed to help a bit."

— PEGGY, *age 48, diagnosed 1996*

"Be prepared for the fact that chemotherapy can bring on menopause either temporarily or permanently. Ask your doctor ahead of time how to deal with hot flashes and the lot."

— BECKY, *age 50, diagnosed 1996*

"I suffered from chemically induced menopause and found that it was helpful at night to keep an extra sleep shirt by the bed. Often I would wake up soaked in sweat from hot flashes and I found it helpful to change into a cool, clean nightshirt."

— RITA, *age 42, diagnosed 1996*

"Chemotherapy is not a picnic. It is not easy, but it is survivable. I had inflammatory breast cancer, underwent an autologous bone marrow transplant, and I'm still here. Remember what your goal is."

— KIMBERLY, *age 41, diagnosed 1993*

Chapter Four

Radiation

"I requested that my treatments
be early in the day so that I
could have the rest of the day to
forget I was a cancer patient."

— RITA, *age 42, diagnosed 1996*

❧

"After I finished chemotherapy, people were quick to tell me what a breeze radiation would be by comparison. Of course these people hadn't had either. I suppose in hindsight, I could say that if chemotherapy were Vietnam, radiation would be like being stationed stateside. You are, however, still in the army!"

— MARGIT, *age 35, diagnosed 1995*

"I was frightened of being tattooed, because I thought it would be painful and disfiguring. It was neither. The tattoos are barely noticeable and I've had mosquito bites that have hurt more."

— LESLIE, *age 32, diagnosed 1996*

"I used Eucerin cream during radiation and had almost no burning."

— ANN, *age 68, diagnosed 1972 & 1991*

"Having my third field radiated during the summer, I needed to protect my skin from the sun up to my collarbone. I wore my scoop neck shirts back to front."

— SHARON, *age 32, diagnosed 1996*

"Since I was taking time off from work anyway, I pampered myself after each radiation treatment by getting together with friends I never had the time to see while I was working."

— MARIANNE, *age 36, diagnosed 1996*

"At the start of my radiation treatments I was just coming off of chemo and was totally bald. By the end of the nearly seven weeks of radiation, my hair had started to grow again. I knew I'd have to go back for the last round of chemo when the radiation treatments were over. I didn't want radiation to end."

— DARIA, *age 34, diagnosed 1996*

"Be certain that the technicians are not mistaking your freckles for tattoos. Mine made the mistake only once, but it was disconcerting enough that I asked them to use a flashlight and double-check for the duration of my treatments."

— MARGIT, *age 35, diagnosed 1995*

"I made an art of arriving with just enough time to undress and change into the hospital gown, with little time to sit and watch and wait for my turn."

— EMILY, *age 42, diagnosed 1996*

"Ask the technicians for an alcohol swab to wipe off the temporary ink marks over the tattoos. It can ruin your bra or blouse if it rubs off. I made a habit of removing the ink and slopping on cream immediately after each treatment."

— PATRICIA, *age 37, diagnosed 1996*

"After Eucerin cream stopped working, I switched to Aquaphor."

— SHARON, *age 32, diagnosed 1996*

"The technicians wanted me to bring in my favorite cassette tape to listen to during my daily treatments. I absolutely refused to do this! The last thing I wanted was to associate a beautiful piece of music with radiation. I let them play their Muzak, and I saved the good stuff for happier times, like the car ride home."

— MARGIT, *age 35, diagnosed 1995*

"I found all of the technicians to be so friendly that I was sad to say good-bye to them when my treatment ended. A month and a half of baring your breast for and sharing your thoughts with people can make you grow quite fond of them."

— DONNA, *age 54, diagnosed 1996*

"I made friends with many of the women that I saw each day in the waiting room of the radiation department. It was nice to have the support of women who understood what I was going through because they were there for the same reason I was."

— LINDA, *age 58, diagnosed 1995*

"I watched every day while we all waited our turn for radiation. All of us talking with each other like we were at some kind of tanning salon or something. I knew that we were all just trying to make the best of a bad situation, but the ease with which we appeared to do this fundamentally bothered me."

— MEG, *age 38, diagnosed 1996*

"I used aloe vera gel on my breast. I kept the gel refrigerated and found it very soothing."

— RONNIE, *age 40, diagnosed 1996*

"I got very tired."

— JOANNE, *age 60, diagnosed 1979 & 1995*

"I got a severe burn from the radiation and had to be put on antibiotics. They tell me that it has nothing to do with how a person tans. There were light-skinned women who didn't burn at all, but I, with my olive complexion, fried like an egg."

— BETH, *age 60, diagnosed 1996*

"I got a bad burn from radiation, so they stopped for a week to let the skin heal a little."

— BARBARA, *age 48, diagnosed 1992*

"I had very little burning at first, but after the fourth week my breast turned very red. It itched and peeled but recovered completely after the treatment ended. You can't even tell I had radiation."

— LINDA, *age 39, diagnosed 1992*

"I had a great deal of tightness in my arm from the radiation. I saw a physical therapist who helped me improve the mobility and deal with the pain."

— MAUREEN, *age 44, diagnosed 1993*

"My nipple turned the same color as my breast (bright red) and when it all began to peel away, it looked like I had no areola. This was frightening. Several weeks after the treatment ended, everything looked normal again."

— SHIRLEY, *age 40, diagnosed 1993*

"I felt like the monkey Virgil, in the movie *Project X*."

— SHARON, *age 32, diagnosed 1996*

"I was fatigued from radiation but I managed to do water aerobics. It aided my strength and self-esteem."

— LORRAINE, *age 56, diagnosed 1993*

"After each radiation session I treated myself to a frozen yogurt."

— GAIL, *age 52, diagnosed 1996*

"Over a six-and-a-half-week period, in the cumulative hours that I spent waiting my turn for radiation, I managed to finish up all of my unfinished knitting projects. I completed 6,100 rads, one sock, one sleeve, two hats, and a sweater vest."

— AMY, *age 46, diagnosed 1996*

"I wore soft cotton undershirts to relieve chafing."

— AUDRIA, *age 42, diagnosed 1996*

"I stopped wearing a bra because it just felt better."

— JUNE, *age 45, diagnosed 1996*

"I drove myself to radiation for the first four weeks but allowed friends to drive me for the last two and a half. I was too pooped to be behind the wheel of a car."

— BOBBY, *age 57, diagnosed 1996*

"I took a nap every afternoon."

— ROBERTA, *age 42, diagnosed 1996*

"After five excisions, radiation was a piece of cake!"

— MARYLEE, *age 52, diagnosed 1995*

"My breast had a small superficial wound from the lumpectomy sutures, which I washed with an antiseptic cleanser called Hibiclens. This helped the area heal enough so that the radiation treatment didn't seem to bother it."

— KIT, *age 47, diagnosed 1996*

"Being alone, isolated in the radiation treatment room, can be frightening. So what I did was count one, two, three, etc., in my head as the treatment was happening to make the seconds pass. I did deep breathing, which helped me relax before and after treatment."

— KIMBERLY, *age 41, diagnosed 1993*

"When finally I was declared ready for radiation, I was extremely fortunate in finding a wonderfully caring radiation oncologist who, with his team of nurses and technicians, made the six weeks of radiation a breeze."

— BARBARA, *age 73, diagnosed 1988*

"The radiation oncologist wanted to do a mastectomy because he said that I would end up too deformed otherwise. I decided not to have a mastectomy. A year later he examined the wrong breast because I looked so good he couldn't tell which was the radiated breast."

— LESLIE, *age 40, diagnosed 1990*

❧

"I remember the first time I saw the patients who were getting radiation for pain control. It scared me to think that this could be me in two years. If you see these people, try to remember that you are a unique person and your outcome will depend on your own set of circumstances. If you happen to be a patient getting radiation for pain control, try to remember that you were once the frightened woman getting adjuvant therapy. Fear can be contagious, but so can hope."

— MARGIT, *age 35, diagnosed 1995*

Chapter Five

Prosthesis

"Get a good prosthesis, even
though it's expensive. My advice is
to smile and wear V necks that
don't quite plunge all the way."

— HOPE, *age 52, diagnosed 1982*

"I bought a prosthesis at Nordstrom, and was fitted by a woman who had a mastectomy as well."

— SUSAN, *age 38, diagnosed 1991*

"I had a prosthesis for eight months, but I was never sure I looked even in it, and was always afraid it would slip away while I was swimming. It only served to convince me that I was a candidate for reconstruction."

— CINDY, *age 42, diagnosed 1993*

"I find that it helps to put the bra on by hooking it on the side, then turning it around and putting the prosthesis in the pocket."

— AMY, *age 44, diagnosed 1995*

"I have used a prosthesis and special bras since the operation. I have taken good care of it and manage to keep it properly aligned to my breast."

— RUTH, *age 74, diagnosed 1984*

"I wore a wig occasionally, but usually wore scarves."

— BETTE, *age 45, diagnosed 1985 &1995*

"I miss my hair but the wig itches so I rarely use it. I use funky scarves, hats, turbans, and cool headwear of various types and combinations. They are always a conversation piece and with big earrings look wonderful! I picked up a great video-tape on how to tie scarves."

— CHRISTY, *age 44, diagnosed 1995*

"I bought an expensive wig locally. It was money well spent—I know I always looked good."

— ANN, *age 68, diagnosed 1972 & 1991*

"I have a prosthesis that can be made to adhere to the body. This has made it easier to go back to running, etc."

— LOIS, *age 50, diagnosed 1994*

"I bought my prosthesis at a surgical supply store. It was very easy for me to adjust to wearing one, although I did forget to put it in my bra a couple of times."

— HELEN, *age 55, diagnosed 1993*

"I got my first prosthesis at the hospital and my second one at a medical supply store."

— ANNA, *age 49, diagnosed 1992*

"I don't wear a prosthesis. Friends joke that I've always worn such baggy clothes that even when I had breasts, you couldn't see my figure."

— CLARA, *age 36, diagnosed 1992*

"Be careful with your wig around the oven. A friend of mine opened her oven, put her head down, and melted the front of her wig!"

— CINDY, *age 40, diagnosed 1994*

"It took me a year to go and buy a prosthesis. I was embarrassed. Finally, I purchased a silicone prosthesis that was too heavy and weighed me down. I eventually settled with a less expensive, more comfortable one."

— BEVERLY, *age 54, diagnosed 1993*

"I went to a place in California, Belle-Amie (see Resources, page 145), which made a mold of my breast before I had my mastectomy. By the time I healed from the surgery, my custom-made prosthesis was ready. It matched my remaining breast quite well in size, color and shape, and even had a nipple and areola. It is an amazingly realistic prosthesis compared to most."

— FRAN, *age 45, diagnosed 1995*

"I had to replace my first prosthesis after two and a half years. Insurance only covers one. After that you're on your own. My advice is to buy a cheap prosthesis to wear with bathing suits and strapless bras, and save the expensive one for your normal wear."

— RAYA, *age 60, diagnosed 1990*

"I purchased a prosthesis from Lady Grace (see Resources, page 145) in the shopping mall. I just couldn't walk into one of those medical supply houses to pick up my breast. I needed an atmosphere that was more relaxed, more normal."

— CINDY, *age 42, diagnosed 1993*

"I bought fake bangs to wear under hats and scarfs. It was more comfortable than a wig and looked quite attractive."

— NICANDRA, *age 40, diagnosed 1994*

"A medical supply house fitted me with a prosthesis that I never liked. Don't let a salesperson tell you what you want. Ask them for guidance, but let your own instincts help you decide what feels the best to you."

— PEGGY, *age 61, diagnosed 1989*

"I wore different wigs for different moods."

— CINDY, *age 42, diagnosed 1993*

"My prosthesis is a 42DD. It feels natural, and looks great!"

— BEVERLY, *age 47, diagnosed 1996*

"Ask your doctor to write a prescription for a scalp prosthesis. You may find that your insurance company will pay for your wig, if it is of medical necessity."

— POLLY, *age 42, diagnosed 1996*

"I ordered a wig, but canceled it before it was styled for me. I wore scarves and hats and coordinated them with new clothes of all colors."

— BEVERLY, *age 54, diagnosed 1993*

"I wear a prosthesis sometimes (Easter, Christmas, special occasions). I think it is a nuisance, but sometimes clothes look better with it on."

— JUANITA, *age 31, diagnosed 1994*

"Don't feel that living with a prosthesis has to be a permanent situation. You can use one for years and get reconstruction later. Personally, I want to recover fully from my cancer treatment before I have any more surgery. By then I may even be comfortable keeping it."

— TAYLOR, *age 38, diagnosed 1996*

"When I went back to work, I wore a wig."

— PEGGY, *age 54, diagnosed 1991*

"I wore a wig to make other people feel more comfortable. In truth, my favorite thing to do was walk around the house totally bald."

— LEE, *age 42, diagnosed 1994*

"After I lost all of my eyelashes I tried false ones. False eyelashes made me look like Bambi, so I thinned them out with hair trimming shears."

— MARGIT, *age 35, diagnosed 1995*

"It's best to make an appointment for a wig while you still have your hair. That way if you want to match your color and style it will be easier."

— RUTH, *age 68, diagnosed 1989*

"If you've lost a great deal of weight from treatment, don't buy a prosthesis until you've stabilized back to your normal weight. You'll save yourself some money."

— KIMBERLY, *age 41, diagnosed 1993*

"Look Good—Feel Better (see Resources, page 145) works with the American Cancer Society to provide classes in cosmetic application, videos and makeup at no charge for women with cancer."

— SUE *age 56, diagnosed 1988*

"I wear no prosthesis and had no reconstruction.
I think of myself as an Amazon warrior with one breast.
I am proud. I am not ashamed of my changed shape."

— SUKY, *age 44, diagnosed 1993*

"Having breast cancer is not the end of the world
provided you find it early enough and you deal with
it. Having a mastectomy is not the worst thing either.
There are good prostheses available today that will
help you be comfortable and look good."

— *Creator of the Barbie doll and the*
Nearly Me Breast Prosthesis Corp.; cofounder of Mattel,
RUTH HANDLER, *age 80, diagnosed 1970*

Chapter Six

Reconstruction

"Immediate reconstruction allowed
me to preserve my body image."

— JULIA, *age 50, diagnosed 1996*

"I always wished that I had the body of an eighteen-year old and the wisdom of an eighty-year-old. Breast cancer gave me both. Now I have a nice flat stomach from the tram flap tummy tuck, a new breast, and the wisdom of experience. Be careful what you wish for!"

— CINDY *age 42, diagnosed 1993*

"My reconstruction was done at the same time as my mastectomy. I was told that this is not always possible to do. Thankfully, I never had the traumatic complication of having to see myself without a breast. It looks different than before, but I am happy with it."

— TINA, *age 54, diagnosed 1996*

"I love my tram flap reconstruction. I feel whole again. It was a long recovery, but it was worth it. I say go for it!"

— CONNIE, *age 41, diagnosed 1985, 1994, & 1996*

"I had no desire to have reconstruction as I did not want further invasion of my chest. I cannot reverse that fact that I had breast cancer. Accepting this has helped me live my life to the fullest."

— BETTY, *age 70, diagnosed 1976 & 1989*

"I had implants. Both leaked and two more were put in. One of those went bad. I would never do it again."

— SALLY, *age 61, diagnosed 1982*

"While I was waiting for my second pathology report to find out whether I would be able to keep my breast, a friend came by to visit me. She gave me one of the best get-well-soon gifts that I ever received. She whipped up her shirt and showed me her beautifully reconstructed breast. Not only did this remove fear of the unknown, but it also gave me hope. Her reconstructed breast was more beautiful than most natural breasts."

— MARGIT, *age 35, diagnosed 1995*

"I had unsuccessful reconstruction and spent two and a half years doing corrective reconstruction. I don't feel it was worth it."

— CHRISTINE, *age 64, diagnosed 1990*

"I have saline implants. Spend the time to learn about what's available. There are lots of shapes and sizes. Don't just let your doctor pick them for you. Get involved."

— PATRICIA, *age 53, diagnosed 1991*

"My implant looks very natural. It was tough surgery but worth it!"

— PAULA, *age 58, diagnosed 1981*

"Be sure that your doctor is a board certified reconstructive surgeon. Be sure to ask what results you can expect, good or bad. There are risks."

— SUSAN, *age 51, diagnosed 1995*

"Always ask the doctors how much experience they have with the procedure you choose. Some techniques are very new. Knowledge will allow you to make an informed decision. Ask questions and read everything you can find!"

— DEBORAH, *age 36, diagnosed 1995*

"I had reconstruction not only for myself, but for my daughter as well. I wanted her to be able to see me with two breasts, so that she wouldn't grow up with the haunting memories that I had from seeing my mother's hollowed chest."

— VIOLET, *age 38, diagnosed 1995*

"Ask to see photographs of finished reconstruction done by your doctor. Most doctors have albums in their offices. Look for pictures of women similar to yourself, both in body type and age, before you consent to surgery."

— LESLIE, *age 26, diagnosed 1995*

"When I started out, I had no idea that a tram flap would mean five surgeries and fifteen months to reconstruct my breast properly. The initial surgery looked horrible. For me the psychological side effects were as difficult as having no breast at all."

— VIRGINIA, *age 52, diagnosed 1994*

"My reconstruction was off to one side so I had one revision. Too much was taken out. Now it's too small. Another revision would mean six more hours of surgery. I'm thinking of having it cut off."

— LINDA, *age 34, diagnosed 1994*

"I didn't have reconstruction. I'm so small that it's not noticeable in clothes."

— PHYLLIS, *age 42, diagnosed 1994*

"I had breast reduction on my other breast at the same time as the tram flap reconstruction."

— KATHLEEN, *age 43, diagnosed 1993*

"I may still opt for reconstruction. It's been years since I had bilateral mastectomies."

— JOANNE, *age 50, diagnosed 1990*

"To celebrate the ten-year anniversary of my date of diagnosis, I gave myself a gift. After ten years of surviving breast cancer, I took time off from work and had a tram flap reconstruction. I now wear my middle aged tummy as a beautiful new breast."

— JILL, *age 45, diagnosed 1986*

"I am very happy with my flap reconstruction. It looks great in clothing and a bathing suit."

— GAIL, *age 41, diagnosed 1994*

"Ask your doctors to put you in contact with other women who have had reconstruction similar to what you are thinking of having. Your doctor can answer medical questions, but the best answers will come from women who have had the procedure themselves."

— MARTHA, *age 32, diagnosed 1996*

"I am a single woman with a single breast. I suppose I give a whole new meaning to the newspaper dating column's term SWF (single white female). I'm pleased to say that this SWF still dates, and has loving, intimate relationships!"

— MOLLY, *age 36, diagnosed 1993*

"There is no sensation in my reconstructed breast, so sexually I feel nothing when it is touched. I do, however, feel sexier having both of my breasts."

— OLIVIA, *age 43, diagnosed 1995*

"I would advise a woman who has to undergo chemo to wait at least one year for reconstructive surgery. I waited three."

— ELLEN, *age 38, diagnosed 1993*

"For me, reconstruction immediately following surgery was a big plus. I had not lost that portion of my body. It was replaced, but not lost."

— RUTH, *age 68, diagnosed 1989*

"Stock up on loose-fitting clothes. After reconstruction, you could have a lot of swelling, and baggy clothes will feel best until the swelling goes down."

— SHELLY, *age 44, diagnosed 1996*

"The stretching I needed was interesting and uplifting compared to the other parts of my treatment. Implants restored my self-confidence."

— MARY, *age 50, diagnosed 1990*

"I found the prosthesis to be a nuisance, so I had reconstruction a couple of years later."

— PATRICIA, *age 52, diagnosed 1985*

❧

"After I was told that my two options were mastectomy or lumpectomy with radiation, I asked about reconstruction. The surgeon was disgusted with my questions and asked me why I would want reconstruction since my childbearing years were over. He felt that I didn't need breasts because I was sixty-five years old. My fourteen-year-old grandson suggested that I tell the surgeon that since he too was past the years of childrearing, he should have his balls removed. It was a crude but effective bit of humor that cheered me up."

— BARBARA, *age 73, diagnosed 1988*

"Even though I had reconstruction, I still need to use a prosthesis because I am a 42DDD."

— ELIZABETH, *age 47, diagnosed 1995*

"I am very pleased with my results. I was back in the gym showing off my newly reconstructed breast just ten days after surgery!"

— DIANNE, *age 31, diagnosed 1995*

"Before I had my reconstruction, which was one year after my mastectomy, I went to a self-help group. I advise other woman to do the same."

— JAQUITA, *age 65, diagnosed 1983*

"I never even considered reconstruction when I heard and saw what it meant. If I had been very young I might have thought differently."

— GENEVIEVE, *age 65, diagnosed 1981*

"I had reconstruction (silicone implant) and have not had any problems."

— SUE, *age 56, diagnosed 1988*

"Many surgeons believe that all women find it psychologically easier to awaken from surgery with reconstruction vs. a mastectomy scar. Women are asked to decide on this while they are under great stress. Unless there are pressing reasons not to delay, the assumption that it is better for *all* women is not necessarily correct. In the service of women thinking they are being given choices, these choices are really being taken away."

— *Senior Social Work Supervisor of Oncology*
for the Beth Israel Deaconess Medical Center, Boston, Massachusetts,
HESTER HILL, *age 48, diagnosed 1993*

Resources

Mail-order contacts for
information, beauty, and comfort

WIG ALTERNATIVES

I WAS IN MY EIGHTH MONTH OF TREATMENT for breast cancer when I knew for certain that women across the country would force this book into becoming a reality. I was shopping for new bedroom slippers at a discount department store, when a woman approached me and asked if I would kindly show her how I had tied the scarf and turban on my head.

She pointed out that her own head of hair was in fact a wig, and that she longed to try a new look, if only she could learn how. We talked for a minute, and I drew diagrams to explain how I had tied my scarf. She thanked me, and I asked her if she'd fill out one of the questionnaires for my book. As we were exchanging addresses, another woman who had overheard us joined in. She too had breast cancer. Within fifteen minutes there were five of us chatting away in the slipper department, all exchanging names, addresses, and advice. One woman even went off into a dressing room to show her reconstructed breast to another woman who was contemplating reconstruction but was fearful of the unknown.

I laughingly said, "Attention Kmart shoppers, there's a breast cancer support group taking place in the slipper department," fully expecting that if this were to be announced over a loudspeaker, half of the store would have appeared!

Wigs are not for everyone. I felt ridiculous in every one I tried on. For ten months I lived in scarves and turbans. On the following two spreads are two of my favorite recipes for dressing up a bald head.

— MARGIT, *age 35, diagnosed 1995*

SIMPLE SCARF AND
TURBAN COMBINATION

This basic turban is a soft cotton cap that will prevent a silk scarf from sliding off a bald head and add a dimension of color. Worn alone, the turban makes a great sleep cap.

▶

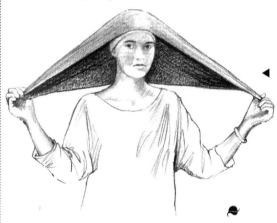

◀ Fold a 34" square scarf in half to a triangle measuring 34" x 34" x 48". Place the long side of the scarf on your forehead, leaving the edge of the turban showing for a touch of color.

Tie at the back
of your neck and
twist length of
ties to ends.

▶

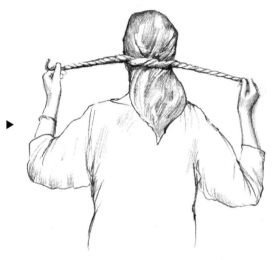

Wrap around your head
and tuck in twisted ends.
◀ Fold up the back of the
scarf, tucking it in at the
back of your neck.

TWO-TONE RIBBON TWIST

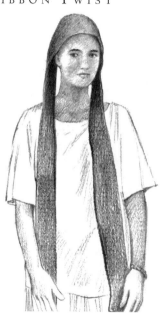

The basic turban is a
soft cotton cap with
long sides. ▶

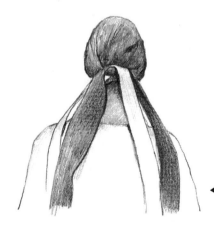

◀ Tie long sides at back of
your neck, folding in one
yard of wide satin ribbon.

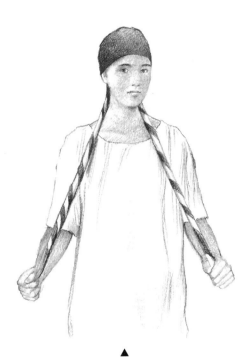

Wrap around your head
and tuck in ends. Try
using different color
combinations . . . pastels
for spring or summer,
black and gold for evening
dressy, red and green for
a Christmas party.

▼

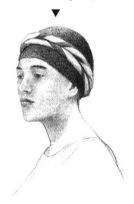

▲

Twist together ribbon
and long sides.

MAIL-ORDER PRODUCTS

Belle-Amie

17815 Sky Park Circle, Suite J, Irvine, CA 92614

800-700-2807 or 714-756-9512

Customized breast prostheses. These are not mail-order prostheses, but are unique for those who can get there and wish to spend the money.

Becoming Inc.

416 West 13th Street, Suite 312, New York, NY 10014

800-980-9085 or 212-989-9788

Silky, sensuous nightgowns that hold prostheses; stylish hats and swimsuits; and elegant wigs.

❧

Bucky

PO Box 31970, Seattle, WA 98103
800-692-8259

Buckwheat hull pillows with soft, fuzzy, warm covers in a wide variety of sizes and colors. The greatest invention for post-op arm comfort!

***Coping* Magazine**

PO Box 682268, Franklin, TN 37068
615-790-2400

Published every other month. Covers issues concerning cancer.

Designs for Comfort Inc.

PO Box 8229, Northfield, IL 60093

800-443-9226 or 847-446-9190

This company makes the Top Cap as well as the Headliner and many other varieties of soft hats and turbans and can provide you with a list of where to buy their products at a store near you. If there is no retailer in your area, they will sell directly to you through the mail.

Feminine Image

3920 North Druid Hills Road, Decatur, GA 30033

800-730-1123 or 404-634-4699

Turbans, lingerie, bathing suits, prostheses, and accessories.

Hair Thoughts from the Heart

1395 E. Dublin-Granville Road, Columbus, OH 43229

800-351-5741 or 614-885-1642

Hats and turbans with a contemporary look.

JHD Enterprise

13619 Mukilteo Speedway, D-5 Suite 396, Lynwood, WA 98037-1606
206-745-0842

Focus on Healing Through Movement and Dance, a fourteen-day-plan audio program designed for all ages and fitness levels, designed for women with breast cancer.

Just in Time, Inc.

PO Box 27506, Philadelphia, PA 19118
215-247-8777

Reversible 100 percent cotton washable headwear, soft hats.

Lady Grace

800-922-0504

Lingerie, swimwear, and prostheses, available at stores on the East Coast and via mail order. Call for a store near you and for mail order.

NutriCology Inc.

400 Preda Street, San Leandro, CA 94577

800-545-9960 or 510-639-4572

Margit's personal choice for hypoallergenic nutritional supplement products.

Paula Young

PO Box 483, Brockton, MA 02403

800-343-9695 or 508-238-0199

Large retailer of affordable, quality, fashion wigs.

Paula's Hatbox

PO Box 935, South Easton, MA 02375

800-332-4287

Hats and accessories.

Perfect Solutions

3030 East Harrison Avenue, Coeur d'Alene, ID 83814

800-296-3098 or 208-664-9112

Stylish hats with detachable human hair bangs. Soft and comfortable.

Salon Perfect Collection

PO Box 4067, S. Hackensack, NJ 07606-4067

800-582-0808 or 201-489-5222

Features the Borghese wig collection, offers color matching service, and arrives fully styled.

Source Cassette Learning Systems

PO Box 6028, Auburn, CA 95604

800-528-2737 or 916-888-7801

A catalog of tapes for stress reduction, relaxation, and healing.

Spenco Medical

PO Box 2501, Waco, TX 76702-2501

800-877-3626 or 817-772-6000

Makers of the Nearly Me breast prosthesis. Will put you in touch with a retailer near you.

Sun Precautions

2815 Wetmore Avenue, Everett, WA 98201

800-882-7860 or 425-303-8585

Features Solumbra sun protective clothing and accessories.

Tresses by Annelise

PO Box 590035, San Francisco, CA 94159-0035

800-988-7377 or 415-583-0269

Classic and contemporary wigs with color matching service.

Organizations with Helpful Information

These are just a few of the many organizations that can help you gather information about breast cancer. The national headquarters are given instead of listing all of their local chapters. By calling or writing to these few organizations one can gather information and help that is close to home as well as e-mail addresses and fax numbers.

American Cancer Society National Call Center

1599 Clifton Road NE, Atlanta, GA 30329-4251

800-ACS-2345

General information, education, and support services including the Reach to Recovery program, Look Good—Feel Better, Making Strides, and other A.C.S.-related programs.

CHEMOcare

231 North Avenue West, Westfield, NJ 07090
800-55-CHEMO or 908-233-1103

A free and confidential service that provides one-on-one emotional support for cancer patients and their loved ones. Patients are matched with trained support people— cancer survivors who have successfully completed surgery, radiation, or chemotherapy.

The Susan G. Komen Breast Cancer Foundation

5005 LBJ Freeway, Suite 370, Dallas, TX 75244
800-I'M AWARE or 972-385-5000

Volunteers work through local chapters and Race for the Cure events to further the Foundation's mission of eradicating breast cancer as a life-threatening disease by advancing research, education, screening, and treatment.

National Alliance of Breast Cancer Organizations

9 East 37th Street, New York, NY 10016

800-719-9154 or 212-889-0606

A network of breast cancer organizations that provides information, education, assistance, and referral to anyone with questions about breast cancer, and acts as a voice for the interests and concerns of breast cancer survivors and women at risk. The NABCO resource list is very comprehensive and available for a small fee or with membership.

❧

National Breast Cancer Coalition

1707 L Street NW, Suite 1060, Washington, DC 20036

202-296-7477

A grassroots advocacy organization that trains and activates all women and men concerned about this disease to effectively focus the public, scientific community, Congress, and the Administration on increasing funding into the cause and cure for breast cancer, improving women's access to high-quality care, and increasing the involvement and influence of women with breast cancer in setting policy.

National Cancer Institute
Cancer Information Service

800-4-CANCER

A hotline with up-to-date information on cancer for patients and their families as well as the general public.

Wellness Community

2716 Ocean Park Boulevard, Suite 1040, Santa Monica, CA 90405

310-314-2555

Provides psychological and emotional support, workshops, lectures, and information, free of charge to cancer patients and family members.

Women's Health Care Educational Network Inc.

PO Box 5061, Tiffin, OH 44883

800-991-8877 or 419-443-1155

A national referral service that will help you locate a retailer near you for all types of women's health care products, focusing on post-breast surgery.

Y-ME

212 W. Van Buren, 4th Floor, Chicago, IL 60607

800-221-2141

Provides information, education, counseling, and free wigs and prostheses for women with financial need if correct size is available and will ship by mail for a small handling fee.

Glossary

Definitions of key words
found in this book, and others
that you may find helpful

Adjuvant therapy: A therapy that aids another method, such as chemotherapy after primary surgery for breast cancer.

Adriamycin: Also called Doxorubicin, a chemotherapy drug sometimes used to treat breast cancer.

Alopecia: Hair loss; a temporary side effect caused by some cancer treatments.

Alternative treatments: Treatments that cover a broad range of healing practices and beliefs. Therapies other than the standard primary treatments of surgery, radiation therapy; and chemotherapy. Examples include acupuncture, massage therapy, herbs.

Anesthesia: Certain drugs or gases used to produce loss of feeling and possibly consciousness.

Antibacterial: An agent that destroys or slows the growth of bacteria.

Antibiotics: Drugs used to treat or prevent infection.

Antidepressants: Drugs used to treat or alleviate depression.

Antiemetics: Drugs used to minimize or prevent nausea.

Antifungal: Drugs that stop the growth of organisms that cause fungal infections.

Anti-inflammatory: Drugs used to minimize inflammation, and the associated heat, pain, and swelling.

Areola: Area of darker skin surrounding the nipple.

Axillary node dissection: Surgical removal of the lymph nodes found in the armpit.

Biopsy: Removal of a sample of tissue to see if cancer is present.

Blood counts: The number of blood cells in a sample of blood.

Bone marrow transplant: Bone marrow previously removed from the patient (autologous) or another person (allogenic) is given to the patient to allow recovery. The use of extremely high doses of chemotherapy to treat cancer destroys the patient's normal bone marrow.

Bone scan: Test used to determine if cancer has spread to the bones. This test can also show other noncancer-related bone changes, such as arthritis.

Calcifications: Small calcium deposits in breast tissue that are detected by mammography. Calcium deposits can occur with breast cancers, but also in benign breast tissue.

Cancer: Disease characterized by uncontrolled, abnormal growth of cells.

Chemotherapy (Chemo): The use of chemicals or drugs to treat cancer.

Clean margins: Term that describes the edge of the tissue that surrounds the removed tumor as being free of cancer.

CMF: Cytoxan, Methotrexate, 5 Fluorouracil. Combination of chemotherapy drugs frequently used to treat breast cancer.

Cytoxan: Cyclophosphamide; a chemotherapy drug frequently used to treat breast cancer.

DCIS: Ductal carcinoma in situ; abnormal cells found in the lining of the duct that have not invaded tissue out of the duct. A breast precancer.

Dehydration: Excessive loss of body fluids.

Duct: A channel in the breast by which milk travels from the lobules to the nipple.

Flap reconstruction: Skin and muscle taken from the back or abdomen to reconstruct a breast after mastectomy.

Frozen section: Tissue that is removed, then frozen, cut into thin slices, and placed on a slide. It is immediately viewed by a pathologist, while a surgeon waits for the information.

Hematoma: Collection of blood under the skin; bruise.

Hemorrhoid: An enlarged vein of the mucous membrane, inside or outside the rectum/anal area.

Hickman: A catheter type device that is placed under the skin and into a major blood vessel. Spares the patient from frequent sticks with needles into arm veins.

Homeopathy: The use of small doses of medicines to stimulate healing, which would produce in healthy people symptoms similar to those of the disease being treated.

Hormones: Chemicals made by glands in the body that can influence the function of certain organs.

Hormone receptor test: Test that determines the amount of hormone receptors (estrogen and progesterone) in breast cancer tissue. If hormone receptors are present, hormones may help the cancer grow, and antihormone treatment may be more effective.

Hot flashes: One of the common symptoms of menopause. Characterized by feelings of warmth, sweating, and sometimes chills.

Immune system: The body systems that fight disease and foreign invaders.

Implant: Substance made of saline (saltwater) or silicone, used by a plastic surgeon to reconstruct a breast.

In situ: Confined to the site of origin. Cancer has not invaded the surrounding tissue.

Infiltrating ductal carcinoma: The cancer has grown outside the duct and into the surrounding tissue.

Inflammatory breast cancer: Rare form of breast cancer in which cancer cells block the lymph vessels to the skin. The skin may appear red, swollen, and warm, and condition may be mistaken for an infection.

Intravenous: Administration of fluids through a vein.

Invasive breast cancer: Most common form of breast cancer that has invaded the surrounding tissue, often forming a lump.

Local recurrence: When cancer reappears in the breast after excision and or radiation, or on the chest wall after mastectomy.

Local therapy: Treatment of the tumor and the area surrounding it with surgery and/or radiation.

Lumpectomy: Surgery that removes the breast cancer and the tissue that surrounds it, without removing the entire breast.

Lymph node: Small glands located throughout the body that filter and destroy bacteria. Cancer cells can spread to the lymph nodes.

Lymphedema: Swelling, usually of the arm or leg, caused by blocked or damaged lymph vessels.

Malignant: Found to be cancerous.

Mammogram: An X ray of the breast.

Mastectomy: Surgery to remove the breast.

Menopause: "Change of life," the span of time during which the menstrual cycle and childbearing ability stop.

Mouth sores: Destruction of cells in the mouth. Mouth sores can sometimes be caused by chemotherapy in the treatment of breast cancer.

Mucous membranes: Surface layer covering cavities that come into contact with air.

Narcotics: Medications used to relieve or treat pain.

Neupogen: Medication that reduces the risk of infection by stimulating the blood system to make white blood cells.

Node negative: Situation in which cancer has not spread to the lymph nodes.

Node positive: Situation in which cancer has spread to the lymph nodes.

Oncologist: Physician who specializes in the treatment of cancer.

Oophorectomy: Removal of the ovaries.

Overall survival: Survival of all patients, with or without disease. Takes into account death from noncancer-related causes.

Partial mastectomy: Surgery that removes the cancer, and part of the surrounding tissue, but not all of the breast tissue.

Pathology report: Analysis of the biopsy, includes the diagnosis and description of the disease.

Phlebotomist: Person who specializes in drawing blood from the vein.

Prognosis: A statement about the likely outcome of disease in a patient.

Prosthesis: Artificial replacement of removed body part.

Protocol: Cancer treatment program; may be experimental.

Rad: Abbreviation for "radiation absorbed dose." A rad is the same as a centigray (cGy), the dose and unit of modern radiation.

Radiation oncologist: A physician specializing in treatment of cancer with radiation.

Radiation therapist: A person who specializes in delivering radiation to treat cancer.

Radiation therapy: The use of high-energy X rays to treat cancer or disease.

Radiologist: A physician trained in performing x-ray procedures and reading X rays.

Reconstruction: The creation by a plastic surgeon of an artificial breast after mastectomy.

Remission: The complete or partial shrinkage of cancer that usually occurs after treatment.

Saline: Saltwater.

Side effect: Unintentional effect of cancer treatment.

Silicone: Synthetic material that is used for breast reconstruction and augmentation.

Stage: Term used to describe the extent of the disease and if the cancer has spread.

Stem cell: The cells that all blood cells develop from.

Stool softener: Medications that treat constipation by preventing the stool from becoming hard and dry.

Systemic therapy: Treatment or drugs that involve the entire body.

Tamoxifen: Antiestrogen used in the treatment of breast cancer.

Tattoo: Small, permanent dots on skin that outline the radiation treatment field.

Third field: The first two fields that treat the breast are angled beams called tangents. A third field may be added to treat the lymph nodes of the clavicle alone, or the clavicle and the axilla.

Tumor: An abnormal growth of tissue, which may be benign or malignant.

Ultrasound: The use of sound waves to visualize structures of the body.

Venous access device: Either a hickman or port-a-cath line. A catheter device that is placed under the skin and into a major blood vessel. May be used to draw blood or give chemotherapy.

WBC: White cell count; the number of white cells in the body that help fight infection.

Zofran: Odansetron, medication used to prevent or treat nausea.

— ELIZABETH A. STAMOS, BN, BS,
Department of Radiation Oncology,
Beth Israel Deaconess Medical Center, Boston, MA

NOTES

Questionnaire

PLEASE TAKE A MOMENT to fill out and mail in this
questionnaire. Your advice may be published in the next
volume and be of great help to other women. Feel free
to expand your answers to a separate sheet of paper. All
personal information is strictly for research purposes and
will remain confidential. THANKS !

1. Name: . . . .

2. Address and phone #: . . . .

. . . .

3. Date of diagnosis: . . . .

4. Age now: . . . .

5. Type of treatment (be specific): . . . .

. . . .

6. If you were married, dating, or living with someone at
the time, in what ways were they, or could they have been,
of support to you? . . . .

. . . .

7. If you had any children at the time, how did you handle
their needs, and in what ways, if any, did they support you?

. . . .

. . . .

8. What other support systems, if any, did you have? . . . . . .

. . . .

. . . .

9. How did you deal with possible side effects and issues associated with various treatments (pain, hair loss, appetite, skin, lymphedema, emotions, work life, health insurance, menopause, sex, relationships, energy level, nausea, self-esteem, etc.)? . . . .

. . . .

. . . .

10. Any advice on surgery, reconstruction, or prostheses?

. . . .

. . . .

11. Any advice on chemotherapy? . . . .

. . . .

. . . .

12. Any advice on radiation? ....

....

....

13. Any mail order products, companies, or services that
you found helpful and would like to recommend? ....

....

....

14. What advice would you give a friend about to go
through breast cancer treatment? ....

....

....

To obtain further copies of the questionnaire or to send in
a completed one, please write to: *Hope Is Contagious*,
Box 3026, Peterborough, NH 03458

❧

YOUR INSIGHTS AND WISDOM are important to us.
If hope is contagious we must continue to spread it
around. Please fill out the questionnaire on the preceding
pages. If it's missing please write us and we'll send you one.
Or feel free just to drop us a line with your comments.

Hope Is Contagious
Box 3026
Peterborough, NH 03458

Acknowledgments

THIS BOOK HAD THE GOOD FORTUNE of being noticed
by literary agent Daniel Strone, of the William Morris
Agency. The attention and care it received was directly due
to Dan's reputation and profound skill. Thank you, Dan,
for giving all of us in the book a chance to be heard.

It took a team of collective talent to put together and
produce this book. Had it not been for the following
people and corporations, neither *Hope Is Contagious* nor I
would be here now. My heartfelt thanks to all of you who
made it possible:

A c k n o w l e d g m e n t s

Dr. Annette Furst (who administers hugs along with Adriamycin), Dr. Pardon Kenney, Dr. Linda Lauretti, Dr. Kathy Mayzel, Janet Rustow, Dr. Norman Sadowsky (the bounty hunter of malignant cells), Dr. Alan Semine, and the entire staff at the Faulkner Hospital, Boston, Massachusetts, who administer medicine with skill and compassion, and who got me through my treatment. Dr. Carolyn Lamb, Elizabeth Stamos, and Judith Hirshfield Bartek of the Beth Israel Deaconess Medical Center, Boston, Massachusetts, Mr. and Mrs. Ian Alexander, Martha Asher, Debra Bard, Ben, Nancy Best, Blue Cross Blue Shield of NH, Patty Cash, The Clark Art Institute, Dr. and Mrs. Gilbert Cogan, Clark Dumont, Kris Earle, Mr. and Mrs. Dan Field, Lyman Gilmore, Roger Goode, Josie Gould, Mr. and Mrs. Roy Hayward, Hiroshi (my link

to the snowflake maker), Aimee Hyatt, Erick Ingraham,
Mr. and Mrs. Court Johnson, Mr. and Mrs. Tom Judd,
Julie Kullgren, Marcela Landres, Nat Lawton, Mr. and
Mrs. Frank Lord, Mr. and Mrs. Norman Makechnie, Michael
Maki DVM, Doreen Means, Doug Mindell, Deborah Morris,
Stephen Muskie, Barbara Pastan, Judi Pettit, Cynthia Porter,
Quad Graphics, Evelyn Rhodes, Samantha, David Serra,
Mr. and Mrs. Steven Siwek, Lida Stinchfield, Margaret
A. Storer Jr., Robert Sullivan, my editor Trish Todd,
Mr. and Mrs. Peter White, Mr. and Mrs. Jay Worthen, Dave
Ziarnowski, practically the entire town of Peterborough,
New Hampshire (seriously!), and the hundreds of women
across the country who authored this book.

Last, I give the greatest of thanks and love to
J Porter, the maker of dreams and my very best friend.

Hopeful

"ONE OF THE POSITIVE SIDE EFFECTS of the treatment is that now that it is over, I can choose to take control of my life again, and seize the day. There are some women who look forward to growing old and planning a long future. I can't live that way. If I plan on growing old I will have everything to lose . . . TIME. But if I cling to the belief that each of my days ahead could be my last, I will have everything to gain . . . TIME! Five or fifty years of days spent in that vein would indeed, for me, be a treasured and happy life!"

— MARGIT, *age 35, diagnosed 1995*

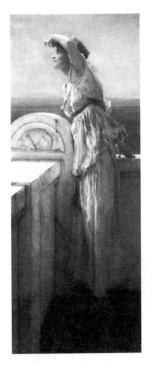

— HOPEFUL, 1909, Oil on Panel, by Lawrence Alma-Tadema, British, 1836–1912